JACQUI LEWIS is a writer, educator, speaker and co-founder of THE BROAD PLACE, a globally focused school sharing ancient knowledge and modern neuroscience, tools and experiences for mindful living. Known for her practical and humorous approach, she leads individual and corporate workshops around Australia and the world.

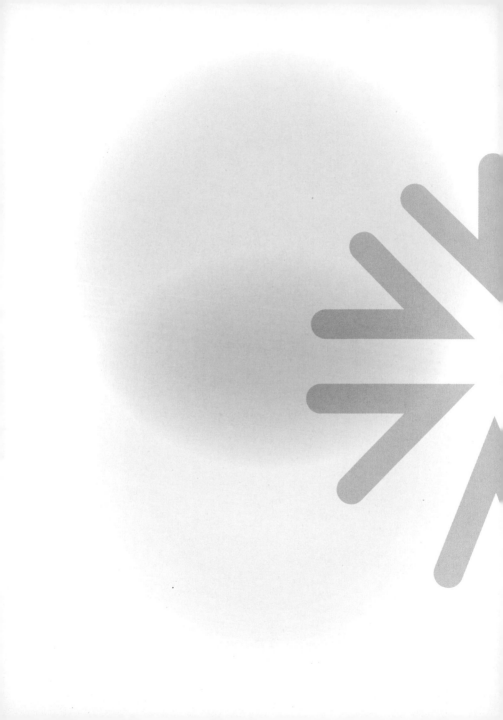

THE

14 day mind cleanse

YOUR STEP-BY-STEP DETOX FOR MORE CLARITY, FOCUS AND JOY

JACQUI LEWIS

chartwell
books

I DEDICATE THIS BOOK

TO ALL OF THE TEACHERS WHO

HAVE HELPED ME ON MY PATH, AS WELL

AS ALL OF THE BROAD PLACE STUDENTS

WHO CONTINUALLY INSPIRE ME WITH THEIR

DEDICATION TO CLARITY, CREATIVITY

AND CONSCIOUSNESS, AND BY LIVING

THEIR MOST ALIGNED LIVES.

CONTENTS

INTRODUCTION

why you will love
a clean, clear mind

'A journey of a thousand miles begins with a single step.'

→ LAO TZU, PHILOSOPHER

These days, the idea of cleansing our bodies has become normalised. Juice cleanses and detox diets are abundantly and enthusiastically adopted. More than ever before, we are taking excellent care of our bodies. There are apps, trainers, nutritionists, physiotherapists, kinesiologists, massage therapists and more to help our bodies be at their best. And I think we can all agree that strong, resilient bodies that are cleansed and healthy – and not filled with toxicity – are great things.

But what about our minds, which govern not just our mental health but also our physical health? How are we cleansing these? What can we do to ensure our minds are in top shape? What about the nutritional value of what we are feeding our minds? And what about the old, outdated crap that's stored in our dusty mental cupboards and emotional storage units?

You know that pristine feeling of clarity when a notion hits you loud and clear, obvious, delicious and full of promise? An idea received when you're rested, grounded and can take action in decisive ways? I believe that being in flow, with crystal-clear clarity and abundant creativity, is as good as the feeling of falling in love. You don't just feel capable, but you thrive. And, delightfully, you're aware of it, which brings about a magnetic energy. It's a mind–body alignment where everything feels possible, rich and full.

When clarity is present, we flow with authenticity and integrity.

So why don't we feel like this all the time? Because we are human. Because we trip, we fall, and we stagnate. But I believe that as long as we can learn from these experiences, they are useful. There are clear, decisive, empowered ways in which we can get out of these ruts and get ourselves back into flow. And each time we do this, we become more resilient and the path becomes clearer. There are always going to be challenges in life: slippery slopes that send us sliding, and mountains that we need to climb. We won't always have the support we might desire, or the energy we might need to navigate the challenges. However, there are techniques we can use to make the entire process a hell of a lot easier – and more joyful. For without happiness and joy, any process – any day of our lives, really – becomes so much harder to get through.

FINDING
the WAY

After being self-employed for over 20 years, as well as being a partner and a mother in a world in hyperdrive, I know all too well the struggles that happen in the modern world: the overwhelm, the anxiety, the slightly dreadful sense of being behind, of tasks piling up, of email inboxes overflowing. There are now so many facets to communicating, so many apps and media, that we are hyperconnected to everyone and everything – but we are also becoming more and more disconnected from ourselves. Add in the competitiveness that seems to appear in every part of our lives now, especially with the comparisons and pitfalls of social media, and it's easy to see why our brains implode at times from too much of everything. But there is a way out, a way to navigate life with less stress and overwhelm, and more clarity and peace.

I founded the school The Broad Place to educate people on being their most aligned, creative, clear selves, and in this book I will share the insights I have discovered by working with people from across Australia, North America, Europe and Asia. I've taught individuals, entire leadership teams, families, corporates, creative types, stay-at-home parents, young children, teenagers, retirees, entrepreneurs and tradespeople. I've had five-year-olds tell me they want to be kinder, and people in their eighties proclaim that you're never too old to be aligned to your higher self. After almost a decade of teaching, I know this to be true:

No matter where you are in life, at some point you will decide that enough is enough and you will want to elevate yourself to be better.

My refined techniques include meditation, practices and rituals that expand consciousness, enhance creativity and increase clarity. They have been tried and tested with so many people living wildly different lives – from so many different age groups and life stages – that I believe they will work for you.

We can be either dragged behind the bus of our lives, or in the driver's seat.

And we can learn not only how to drive, but also how to drive with excellence, to cope with tricky driving conditions and to stay cool under pressure. This is not some mystical ideal only attainable by monks who live in Himalayan caves, removed from the world. This is for anyone and everyone who wants to be their kindest and most compassionate and caring selves. The key is that it has to start with us. Too often we are focused on fixing everyone else's lives. The 14 Day Mind Cleanse is a program for *you*, so you can be your clearest and most grounded self – this also helps you to be of better service to others. And guess what? They're invested in this, too. When you show up with more joy and resilience, everyone around you benefits.

We are going to tackle this in two ways: by introducing things that will calm, soothe and ground you, bringing you more clarity; and by reducing or even pausing things that make you feel foggy, stressed, anxious and tired.

Let's get clear on what the 14 Day Mind Cleanse is:

> A two-week program to reset your mind. Just like the clothes you wear, your mind gets worn out, muddied up and tired. In this program, we'll hit refresh, running your mind through a hot wash and rinse cycle. It's like taking a huge basket of dirty clothes, washing them, letting them dry in the sun with a gentle breeze, and then inviting them back in, fresh, warm and restored.

> A way to empower yourself with a philosophy to cope with modern life, giving you the techniques to hit reset on your mind whenever overwhelm hits.

The 14 Day Mind Cleanse is *not* a wellness project. It does not instruct you to make green smoothies, wear activewear all day long or journal on a beach to achieve wellbeing.

WHAT
is INVOLVED?

The 14 Day Mind Cleanse is a step-by-step program to reset your mind. The first week involves learning one new building-block technique each day, starting with a beginners' meditation, and adding each new building block to your daily routine. By Day 7, you will have a program of seven daily techniques that will help you build clarity. If you'd like to take things further, each day also includes an optional extension to try, such as setting intentions. The second week is a deep mind cleanse, using all seven techniques every day plus journalling.

The 14 Day Mind Cleanse is not a lightning-bolt process, but a daily transformation over two weeks. Here are some of the things we will be working on:

> cleansing your mind with a daily meditation practice

> setting the stage for better, deeper sleep with an hour of powering down before bed

> learning to stop multi-tasking and be more mindful

> starting your day with a personalized morning ritual

> banishing 'busy' by prioritizing tasks and reframing your language

> curating and improving what you feed your mind

> increasing your happiness by 'joy-riding'

16

The 14 Day Mind Cleanse is incredibly easy to follow. This is deliberate because, if you're anything like my students, when you're in a rut or overwhelmed, you want solutions that work and you want them now. You don't have the time or the inclination to take a huge sabbatical to 'find yourself', or to listen for hours and hours to workshops and seminars just to get results. I want you to be able to pick up this book on a Sunday night, when the week ahead is looming, and turn your whole week around, starting first thing Monday morning.

You might have withdrawal symptoms as you reduce addictive habits such as overusing your mobile phone and other technology, creating unnecessary busyness and complaining about everything. But you must remember that this book will be a key building block for you to **live with more clarity, kindness, flow and creativity.**

At the end of the 14 days, you'll know through actual practice which techniques work for you. Then you can decide what to keep up and what to let go of. You might continue to use some techniques each day, others once a week. You might want to repeat the 14 Day Mind Cleanse every six months, each season or once a month – or whenever you feel a little wobbly in life. It's totally up to you.

17

SO WHAT'S GOING TO HAPPEN
over the next two weeks?

You will explore the mind–body connection to understand how they affect each other.

You will employ mental exercises to reduce stress and increase your clarity and happiness.

You will meditate daily for a fitter, stronger mind.

You will have an hour of digital disconnection every day.

You will learn to focus your attention on one thing at a time.

You will create a custom morning ritual for more grace in your day.

*You will understand how
to reframe your perspective
on busyness.*

. . . .

*You will gain clarity on the
information with which you
are nourishing (or poisoning)
your mind.*

. . . .

*You will become conscious
of negative thought patterns,
and work on reframing them
with more helpful thinking.*

. . . .

*You will finish the two weeks
refreshed, with a clear mind
and renewed values.*

. . . .

BEFORE YOU BEGIN

understanding the mind–body connection

'Training your brain to manage stress won't just affect the quality of your life, but perhaps even the length of it.'

→ AMY MORIN, PSYCHOTHERAPIST

Over the next two weeks, you are going to focus on high-quality thinking and mindfulness. This means becoming self-aware – being fully conscious of the present and what you are doing in this moment. Right now! Our minds govern so much of what happens in our bodies, and we tend to flit between the past and the future constantly, rarely absorbing what is happening in the present. But the truth is that the present is all we have.

How do we become self-aware? Simply by improving the way our minds work, which involves rewiring the neural pathways in our brains. It used to be believed that once the thought patterns in the brain – or 'wiring' – were set, we couldn't change them. However, through the latest studies in neuroscience, we now know that the brain is actually malleable (commonly referred to as 'plastic'). Neuroplasticity is the brain's ability to change through learning.

Once a thought is created in the mind, the body instantly responds; these reactions are stored in our nervous systems. On average, we experience anywhere between

80,000 and 90,000 thoughts a day. Some scientists say it is up to 120,000 thoughts a day! These are constantly and instantaneously affecting the 37 trillion cells we have in our bodies. Put simply, it's extremely important to start being aware of the quality of our thoughts and the impact they are having on our physical and emotional health.

Our minds are incredibly powerful, and we need to take care of them in order to be at our best.

This starts with cleansing – clearing a little time during which the brain has a tiny break from the exterior world barging in each day. It's where we can stem the tide of emails, notifications, TV and social media. We can also work on being more present and more attentive.

Over the next 14 days, you'll become more mindful of your thinking patterns. You'll combine high-quality thinking with positivity, self-compassion and kindness, applying the very best of both ancient practice and modern knowledge. But before we begin, let's go over some important points about how the body is linked with the mental capacity of the mind and the physical structure of the brain.

Welcome to your
LIMBIC SYSTEM

Deep inside your brain, just above the brain stem, a complex set of structures can be found. Known as the limbic system, it is made up of the hypothalamus, the amygdala and a number of other structures (such as the thalamus). In addition to being in charge of our emotional lives, it is also where memories are formed. It gathers important information that is then communicated to the rest of the body through the autonomic nervous system or the pituitary gland (called the master of all glands, as it controls the hormones).

Although the hypothalamus is small, it is crucial for helping the body to maintain a state of balance (homeostasis). It constantly calibrates all of the body's systems, with the goal of returning these systems to a set point. This is how we maintain a safe core temperature regardless of whether the room is cool or warm. It's also why we shiver or experience a deeply cold feeling when we suffer heat stroke – our hypothalamus is trying to bring down our body temperature. The hypothalamus is also involved with blood pressure and gut health, as well as the sensations of hunger, pain, thirst, anger and pleasure, and sexual drive.

The amygdala consists of two small, almond-shaped masses sitting on either side of the thalamus. This is the kitchen in which our primal reactions are cooked up. It is stimulated during times of stress, helping us to become aggressive when absolutely necessary. When we are in dangerous situations, it allows us to have quick and instantaneous reactions – the renowned fight or flight response. In experiments where the amygdala has been removed, subjects cease to react to fear and they also become completely indifferent to life-threatening situations and sexual desire.

Much of the information gathered by the limbic system is communicated to the body by the autonomic nervous system, which is made up of two parts: the sympathetic nervous system and the parasympathetic nervous system.

The sympathetic nervous system (SNS) accesses a variety of body areas. Its main job is to physically prepare us for the vigorous activities – such as running from danger, diving into deep water and defending ourselves against violence – associated with our fight or flight response. When we are faced with a threat, the SNS sends a shout-out to the adrenal glands to rapidly release adrenaline into the bloodstream, our cortisol (stress hormone) levels rise, and we are ready to put up our best fight or to run away quickly.

The parasympathetic nervous system (PNS) brings our bodies back into balance after the effects of the SNS have been utilised and are no longer needed. The PNS manages and maintains blood pressure, carbon dioxide levels, adrenaline production and more. What's interesting to note is that when we meditate, the PNS turns on. From here, healing and repair can take place at a very deep level.

Basically, the autonomic nervous system involves a very tight procedure. Something happens to us, and our brains process the emotion associated with it. A message is sent to our SNS, there is a physical reaction, and then our bodies rebalance thanks to the PNS. This is a very natural and necessary process, but it is designed to be used only in short, infrequent bursts. When it is called upon frequently, health problems can arise.

WHEN FIGHT OR FLIGHT
goes awry

The fight or flight response is our basic reaction to a threat: do we attack what's in front of us, or do we run away? Two other responses are often also distinguished: freezing and fawning (surrendering). All four responses are in-built to instinctively protect us from bodily harm.

Following an event, nerve cells rapidly begin firing and chemical releases start to flood the body, and we are now physically and psychologically prepared for fight or flight. Today, we don't often find ourselves needing to run from a tiger or fight a territorial caveman, yet modern life, traffic snarls, deadlines, financial worry, pandemics and so on are causing us to spend a lot of our time in this state of fight or flight. When we experience these triggers, our bodies release adrenaline and cortisol. Our respiration rate increases, digestion slows and our muscles tense.

In this state, we start to see everything around us as a threat. Unfortunately, this process skips past our rational mind and our higher selves, the place where we are calm, grounded and more able to make conscious and effective decisions. As our thinking narrows and our perspective is distorted, our brains are being given the signal to seek out and focus on any potential risk. We are now seeing the world through the lens of fear. And as deadlines and traffic continue to be part of our lives, we continue to view the world in this way.

If we spend a lot of time with these stress hormones and chemicals circulating around our systems, we leave ourselves wide open to disease and poor general health.

Currently in Australia, cases of high blood pressure, diabetes, poor gut health, low immunity, hormonal imbalance and autoimmune disease are higher than ever, and this has been linked to our inability to effectively metabolize the amounts of stress hormones and chemicals constantly in our bloodstreams. With regard to emotions, there are high rates of depression, anxiety, stress, reduced self-worth and lack of ambition; many people also find it difficult to relate to others and be compassionate.

We are spending more and more of our time in a physiological state that makes it almost impossible to cultivate positivity and to see the forest for the trees. It's important to realise that the pressure of modern living is not a bad thing – we are very adaptable, creative beings who have constructed a fast-paced world in which we aim to thrive and get ahead. It's just that in constantly wanting to do more and be better, we've become caught up in a loop where our bodies are struggling to survive. This loop has become much more of a habit than a necessity to function at our best.

When we are overwhelmed, stressed, sick, depressed or burned out, we can't think with clarity – so we stay stuck.

When we are grounded, confident and stable emotionally, we are inclined to take a step back and see the bigger picture of life in general and our place in it. This is one of the key reasons why meditating daily is vital. It allows us to gain greater perspective and motivation, and to re-examine our beliefs, values and goals. Our bodies start to recalibrate, rebalance and realign to a restful, peaceful state. In this state, we become dynamic, clear, creative and focused, and we are guided towards the things and people that support this new and natural way of being. This also means that in moments of true crisis – such as when a firefighter has to run into a burning building, or a parent goes to extreme lengths to save a child – we are primed and ready, rather than exhausted from all of the stress chemicals in our bodies.

Often, what we do to counteract these states of stress and disease is counterproductive. We long for the end-of-day wine, or we eat large amounts to distract ourselves. Our fight or flight response has been activated, yet we can't attack or flee from most of our modern-day 'threats' – so instead we become aggressive, sad, worried or hyperactive. Unfortunately, all of these responses are actually pointless when it comes to our survival. Imagine if we started punching the wheel and tearing apart our car as we sat in a traffic jam, or we got out and ran away, leaving the car in the middle of the street? I'm sure you would agree that these kinds of responses are not beneficial to our emotional, psychological and spiritual evolution.

If we are able to shine some light on our automatic responses, becoming aware of the times we tend to go into fight or flight unnecessarily, this will help us to stop engaging in it.

If we are able to understand these very human responses and create some distance from them, then we can create a much more stable mind and body. We can even begin to use the fight or flight response to our advantage. For example, when we are launching into a new event and everything is moving quickly, we can harness the sharpened mental reactions and surge of energy to be productive. And when we are in situations outside of our control or when a state of calm is more productive, we can choose not to engage in the psychological stimulus that kickstarts our fight or flight response. The techniques I am going to outline within the 14 Day Mind Cleanse will help you transform your responses, nervous system and thinking through awareness and practice.

So now that you have a basic understanding of what's happening in your brain, mind and body, let's get started!

WEEK 1

build skills

'There is only one corner of the universe you can be certain of improving, and that's your own self.'

→ ALDOUS HUXLEY, AUTHOR

What a sensational time it is to begin your 14 Day Mind Cleanse! Before we start, let's take a moment together to get clear on what it is you wish to experience throughout the two weeks, and how committed you are. I also have some tips that will help you through this process.

Creating new habits can be a neurological challenge when we have so many old, redundant habits ruling our days.

The key is to acknowledge that transformation takes time, as well as motivation, inspiration and discipline. We can get frustrated along the way, we can become tired of rewiring our beliefs and behaviors, and we need a lot of care for ourselves, from ourselves. So show kindness and compassion towards yourself.

This first week in particular – as you learn something new, and adopt a fresh technique every single day – can be very exciting. At times, it can also be overwhelming for your brain. This is why we have one week to adopt the new techniques, and then another week to really absorb them. Expect that challenges might arise and discipline might waver, and acknowledge right now that you're a human being doing your best – sometimes things don't go exactly to plan. Of course, I recommend really applying yourself, but if you're also flexible and you go gently, you will learn as much from the 'mistakes' as you do from 'getting it right'.

To begin, I recommend jotting down a few key points about why you are undertaking this 14 Day Mind Cleanse. Then ask yourself how you wish to feel at the end of the two weeks. What kind of commitment are you ready to make to bring more clarity into your life? And what are you really prepared to pause during this next fortnight that you know is already undermining your clarity and decision-making?

Good luck, and I'll be with you every step of the way!

Week 1 overview

Each day you will learn a new technique and add it to your routine. This is what you will do each day during Week 1:

DAY 1 **mind cleanse meditation**

DAY 2 **mind cleanse meditation**
power down hour

DAY 3 **mind cleanse meditation**
power down hour
reduce mashing

DAY 4 **mind cleanse meditation**
power down hour
reduce mashing
morning ritual

DAY 5 **mind cleanse meditation**
power down hour
reduce mashing
banish busy

DAY 6 **mind cleanse meditation**
power down hour
reduce mashing
morning ritual
banish busy
mind nutrition

DAY 7 **mind cleanse meditation**
power down hour
reduce mashing
morning ritual
banish busy
mind nutrition
joy ride

DAY 1

mind cleanse meditation

get mindfit with a daily practice

'Meditation will not carry you to another world, but it will reveal the most profound and awesome dimensions of the world in which you already live.'

→ HSING YUN, ZEN MASTER

$\rightarrow$ *mind cleanse meditation*
power down hour
reduce mashing
morning ritual
banish busy
mind nutrition
joy ride

Welcome to your first day of the 14 Day Mind Cleanse! Today, I'll introduce the foundation for your crystal-clear mind: **meditation**.

Before diving in, it's important to remember that not all meditation is designed and practiced the same way. Nor do all meditation techniques achieve the same results. Most people think meditation is a blanket term for 'less stress', or imagine some kind of bliss-filled bubble that they will enter on closing their eyes – and they are then shocked to discover that this isn't the case when they attempt meditation! So many people say they've tried meditation but it 'didn't work'. I counter that they just haven't found a technique that suits their particular mind and body.

I'm going to first address meditation as a practice, and then teach you the Mind Cleanse Meditation. One of the most frustrating things I have found is that meditation books often say how great meditation is, but they don't share any actual techniques. I'm going to teach you a beginners' meditation practice, which you can start using immediately.

the MEDITATION TRIO

There are three primary types of meditation: contemplative, concentration and transcending.

CONTEMPLATIVE TECHNIQUES *are where **your mind is taken on a journey**, such as by listening to a guided meditation, or you are deeply considering something, such as gratitude. Examples include using the Headspace app, watching a YouTube video or following a guided meditation at the end of your yoga class.*

CONCENTRATION TECHNIQUES *are where **you focus your mind**, perhaps by chanting repetitively, watching your breath or focusing on one part of the body. Examples include Vipassana and Zazen practices.*

TRANSCENDING TECHNIQUES *are where **you work gently with a mantra to allow the mind to naturally and effortlessly transcend thought** and access deeper states of consciousness. Examples include Integrated Meditation, Transcendental Meditation, Vedic Meditation, Deepak Chopra's Primordial Sound Meditation and the Mindfit Meditation that I teach at The Broad Place.*

I have practiced and taught all three primary meditation styles for a long time. They work well in different situations, for different people with different lifestyles. I find that a guided meditation (from the contemplative camp) is perfect for a one-off experience, perhaps as part of a retreat or corporate program. It works well when there is a clear understanding of what the meditation is trying to achieve (such as deep relaxation, true forgiveness or the accessing of inner wisdom), partnered with a beautifully executed meditation experience. The thing about guided meditations is that you need to be led by either a teacher or an app (which means you're connected to technology). You also need a calm, quiet, Zen-like environment.

Trying to do a guided meditation every day can be complicated. You may get bored if you are doing the same meditation over and over again, and this can lead to a never-ending quest to find new meditations if you want to make this a daily practice. Most people get bored after a few weeks, then frustrated, then stop altogether. Let's face it: having someone's voice in your head every day when you're trying to disconnect from your own incessant inner voice – and when you also have the world chattering at you constantly – doesn't make for the most appealing approach to meditation.

Throughout history, guided meditations have often been done in monasteries and ashrams as part of a much larger daily meditation tradition, which is very different from how we might fit in the practice now, in between phone calls and emails and while juggling work and home life. Concentration meditation techniques are usually done in residential retreat-style settings. For example, a ten-day Vipassana program of silence – along with physical and emotional austerities – is the initial training, which is then followed up with a daily hour-long meditation practice both morning and evening. These are quite intensive and challenging techniques for today's busy, overwhelmed mind.

43

MEDITATION
for the
MODERN WORLD

All meditation techniques are valid and have their place. What is frequently missed, though, is a consideration of *why* you want to meditate and what you want to receive from your practice, while factoring in your lifestyle. How much time can you reserve to meditate? Do you have a quiet time and place to do it, or will you be meditating whenever and wherever you can grab a moment?

Most of the students I teach are time-poor, have a lot on their plates at work and at home, and feel that meditation is beyond them. My aim is to introduce them to techniques that evolve their minds and consciousness but also fit into their lifestyles. Because of this, I usually teach transcending meditation techniques.

*Your overworked mind needs a 'defrag',
a reprieve and a reset from the action
it endures all day long.*

A mantra-based transcending technique doesn't require a quiet space – it can be done anywhere – and it is luxurious because you can sit comfortably rather than in a complex yoga position. It's a resilient, wonderful practice that can be incorporated into your life in a variety of ways.

Now, there is a difference between the meditation technique I'll teach you in this book and the other meditation practices I teach in person: Mindfit Meditation and Integrated Meditation. Mindfit Meditation is an intermediate-level practice of meditating once daily with universal intentional mantras for 15 minutes, and it is taught during a ten-day course. Integrated Meditation is a more advanced practice that involves receiving a special personalized mantra during a live interactive course in which you meditate for 20 minutes twice daily. I believe that Integrated Meditation is the world's most effective meditation technique. It's a total game-changer. Tens of thousands of people all over the world have learned this ancient technique to increase their creativity, intelligence, physical health and happiness.

In this book, I am going to share with you a beginner-level style of meditation with a mantra to get you up and running: the Mind Cleanse Meditation, which you can do for ten minutes once a day. Just like the other two mantra-based techniques, Mind Cleanse Meditation is not about creating airy-fairy meditation episodes, but about supporting your mind and body through deep relaxation and rest, so you can be happier and optimise your days.

We are not trying to create an 'experience' with the Mind Cleanse Meditation. You'll find that no two meditation sittings are the same: some are rough as hell, while others are graceful and easy. Don't get too caught up in this. We are meditating because of the overall impact it has on our lives, not just the effect it has during the period we sit with our eyes closed. When my students say that they're clearer and more focused, productive, creative and emotionally resilient – as well as less stressed, anxious and tired – as a result of their meditation practice, they mean in their days and in their lives as a whole, *not* during the time they actually sit to meditate! So drop all of your expectations, and let's begin.

PREPARING *for* *your* MEDITATION

Let's get the foundations for your daily practice sorted. You will need to find ten minutes every day to meditate. Some people love to do this first thing on waking, sitting up in bed. Others like to stretch, have a cup of tea and then meditate. Many people prefer to refresh themselves with their Mind Cleanse Meditation in the afternoon, as a productivity booster. Just don't do it too close to bedtime. Meditation can sometimes put you in a more deeply restful state than a nap, so in the same way you wouldn't have a nap too close to bedtime, you shouldn't meditate and then try to go to sleep.

It doesn't matter when you do it, but make sure you DO IT. You can't see the benefits without actually sitting to meditate, in the same way you can't get fit without actually exercising (I wish!). And just as with going to the gym, you will see the benefits over time, accumulating outside of your 'work-out sessions'.

You don't need a magical, quiet space to meditate.

If you have one on hand, by all means go for it. But many people meditate in their parked cars, on the bus, at work, on a park bench, sitting up in bed with kids sleeping next to them – you get the idea.

It's not necessary to practice at the same time each day in the future, but I recommend that for the next 14 days you find a similar time of day to sit. Mark it in your calendar and set an alarm to remind you, so you can be sure to get it done.

Preferably, don't use a timer during the meditation. But how do you know when your ten minutes are up? At first, you'll probably check your watch a few times, and that's okay. If you have an A-type personality, you might want to start with setting a timer just to calm yourself down. However, in the long term, we drop timers and become independent of the need for tech to meditate. During the meditation, ensure that your phone is on silent or, better still, on airplane mode. Avoid checking your phone, emails or social media as soon as you sit to meditate. It distracts you from meditating peacefully, and you'll soon lose your allocated meditation time.

Mind Cleanse Meditation is not a stillness competition. So if you need to shift about, scratch or sniff, do so! You'll want to sit up in a comfortable position, with your back supported and your head free (so don't lean your head on a wall). Don't do your Mind Cleanse Meditation lying down, either – this position turns on the sleep receptors in the brain. Sit on the floor with your legs crossed or straight out; even better, sit on a chair.

your
MANTRA

You're going to be meditating with a mantra – a simple, universal word that will likely make you wonder: 'How the hell can this possibly work?' Trust me, do this ten-minute meditation for the next 14 days, and you'll soon see the benefits. The key thing is not to be forceful with the sound of the mantra. You are going to be gentle, repeating your mantra softly in your mind, so it sounds like a breeze blowing through the trees. Does that mean your mind will stay serene? Heck no. As soon as you begin repeating the mantra, your body will start releasing stress and fatigue as you move into deeper states of rest, which will then make your mind active. This is why you have the mantra: it's like an anchor in a stormy sea. You don't want to cling to your anchor as if you're drowning; just gently return to it in the sea of thoughts, outside noises, bodily sensations and myriad experiences while meditating.

You're not trying to banish thoughts. Just keep gently returning your focus to your mantra whenever thoughts pop up. And believe me, you will have LOTS of thoughts. That's totally okay. We couldn't stop our minds from thinking even if we tried. It would be like trying to stop your heart from beating. Don't use your mantra to bat your thoughts away, or increase the volume of your mantra to combat noisy thoughts. Consider your thoughts as fish in the sea, swimming about. Just stay with your mantra, going with the flow as the thoughts swim around you. You can't mess it up. Feel antsy and agitated? That's good: stress is leaving your body. Feel tired? That's fine, too. Meditation releases fatigue. Something good is ALWAYS happening. You just need to keep meditating to get the results.

Now, you're not going to chant this mantra, or yell it out. And you're not going to hold a rhythm for it, or make it do anything tricky. You're going to use it softly, slowly and effortlessly. Your mind will do all sorts of strange things in and around it, and you'll drift off a lot. Just return to it again … and again … and again. This is the process: being soft and gentle, and going with the flow of whatever is happening rather than fighting it with frustration. Eventually, you'll become very good at letting it go. The mantra will drift off on its own and your mind will transcend, and other times you will feel so deeply relaxed that you will just let it go and have a tiny pocket of silence. This won't last long, as a stream of thoughts will soon barge in, and then it's time to reintroduce your mantra.

So you now have a ten-minute window in which to work with a mantra. You know how to sit, you know what to do, so what is this mantra? A note about mantras: there are a ton of them. They mean different things, and also do different things. When you learn Mindfit Meditation, you choose from a menu of mantras, depending on what you're looking for from that meditation. When you learn Integrated Meditation, you receive a personal mantra from the Vedas, an ancient body of knowledge from India. What I am going to give you now is a single anchor point for your mind to remember and gently return to when thoughts arise.

Your mantra is the word
ONE.

'One' can represent the harmony of the universe, or the first and distilled of all the numbers; it can also be a reminder that your mind and body are united. It really doesn't matter what 'one' means to you, as we are not using the left, analytical hemisphere of your brain during meditation. This is the side that wants to break everything apart and understand; it's the linear, list-making side. Meditation is going to optimise the right, lateral, creative side of your brain. The mantra 'one' will provide your mind with something to focus on during your meditation, so that other things can take place. Just sit down and go for the ride!

I wish you the best of luck as you start your two-week journey to a clearer, calmer, steadier mind. But don't forget: meditation is not just for the next 14 days. On completing the 14 Day Mind Cleanse, you can continue with your daily ten-minute Mind Cleanse Meditation to enhance your mental fitness. To take your practice further, you can sign up for an in-person or online meditation class at The Broad Place or elsewhere. Meditation is truly the cornerstone of a life well lived, so dedicate the time to it and you will reap so many benefits.

MIND CLEANSE MEDITATION

Starting today, do a ten-minute Mind Cleanse Meditation every day at approximately the same time. Here is a step-by-step guide to your daily meditation practice:

1 Select a suitable place to meditate.

2 Put your phone on silent, or better still on airplane mode.

3 Sit in a comfortable position, with your back supported and your head free.

4 Softly repeat the mantra 'one' to yourself. Whenever thoughts pop up (and they will), gently return to your mantra.

5 Continue for ten minutes.

52

EXPERIMENT WITH MINDFULNESS

Mindfulness — or being present — is the output of a great meditation practice. There are some extra layers you can engage with, though, to train a fractured mind to be more present, and I will outline some here for you to try.

Walk with Presence

Kinhin is a meditative practice from Zen Buddhism that involves walking with absolute presence. It is done slowly — the slower the better — so you can be present for every single movement and breath as you go. You can do it around your home, or in a garden. When you begin, it can feel like you're in a slow-motion film (and, honestly, it can look a little weird!). So perhaps the best place to start is at home. Traditionally, it is done in the meditation hall or garden of a retreat.

As you walk slowly, you will begin to notice every muscle in your feet, your legs and your shoulders, the way your hips and pelvis support you, and the way your spine ripples as you move. Each breath becomes deeper and slower, and the way your lungs are filled and emptied becomes very present. It's a truly beautiful thing to do, especially as we often take walking and breathing for granted. One keeps us mobile, while the other keeps us alive! Taking some time to engage with these two important actions on a deeper level can have a profound effect on your gratitude and your presence, and also on how you move through your day. A period of five or ten minutes is plenty of time to do Kinhin when you first begin.

Shower Mindfully

We are frequently distracted while showering, either because we are rushing or because we are just standing there, numbing ourselves. Bring about a mindful and peaceful awareness, and try showering as a meditative experience. Before you stand under the water, feel how dry your skin is. Then become aware of the water temperature as it first hits your skin – do you get goosebumps? Keep checking in as you shower and your skin is calibrating to the water temperature. Then embrace the aroma of the body wash you use. Are there any other scents in the bathroom? Watch the steam rise and shapeshift. As you finish the shower, what sensation do you have once you turn off the water? When your skin touches the towel? And how do you feel when you are completely dry? As we shower daily, we can dive into more nuances as we go along.

This is a wonderful way to train our minds to become more present every day, and to really enjoy the process of a daily habit that is so often overlooked for its potential joy.

Watch a Sunrise

The sun is called *Surya* in Sanskrit, and a way to greet it is by saying 'Jai Surya', which essentially means 'Hello sun'. A wonderful meditative practice is to watch the sunrise from beginning to end – from the moment the sun peeks over the horizon until that ball of light is completely in the sky. Sit or stand and relax into your body, and then practice patience as you view this extraordinary show. Note that the sun is not actually 'rising', as we call it, but that we are rotating on earth. Taking a few minutes to observe this process with utter presence can bring about a deep sense of joy, wonder and awe. (If you're not a morning person, then try watching the sunset instead!)

55

DAY 2

power down
hour
create
the break
your mind
needs

'Sometimes
you have to
disconnect to
stay connected ...
We've become
so focused on
that tiny screen
that we forget ...
the people right
in front of us.'

→ REGINA BRETT, AUTHOR

mind cleanse meditation
→ power down hour
reduce mashing
morning ritual
banish busy
mind nutrition
joy ride

We are more connected now than at any other time in human history. Our access to information is unprecedented, and technological advances abound. Yet more people feel disconnected, stressed and anxious than ever before. All of this is literally changing our brains.

In 2017, Deloitte surveyed 4150 British adults about their mobile-phone habits. Overall, 38 per cent thought that they were using their smartphone too much. Among 16- to 24-year-olds, that number rose to more than 50 per cent. Habits such as checking apps in the hour before we go to sleep (79 per cent of us do this, according to the study) or within 15 minutes of waking up (55 per cent) may be taking a toll on our mental health.

Now, let's be honest. I researched and wrote this book on a computer, and I will promote it online through social media. Personally, I adore modern technology. But I can't deny its impacts. It's altering human physiology, and not necessarily for the better.

The solution isn't giving up technology. It's giving your tired, strained brain a little break from it. It's about daily digital disconnection.

The Power Down Hour
is one simple change that will
help you to feel calmer and more
relaxed. Think of it as a tiny
brain holiday each and every day.
Trust me, the results will be
incredible.

POWER DOWN HOUR

Starting tonight, during the hour before you go to bed, put all tech away. It's a much-needed little digital break for the 60 minutes before you go to sleep. This means switching off your mobile phone, TV, computer, laptop, tablet, MP3 player . . . all of it. You can do other things in this hour if you like — read a book, have a bath or shower, talk to family members or flatmates, perform a face-cleansing ritual, light candles — things that help you wind down, be present and relax. Ultimately, they're the things we did BEFORE we had technology, which wasn't that long ago!

Too often we are utterly distracted by other people's views and the world as a whole. This takes away from our ability to become our own compass to guide how we show up in the world. We have to disconnect from technology and social media to really create a connection to our true selves.

This disarmingly simple technique is actually quite hard to do. The Power Down Hour can be a bit challenging to fit in, and it is easily forgotten or left too late. So set an alarm for ten minutes before you want to begin powering down at night. Give your brain the break it deserves! If you want to take this to the next level, I suggest a second Power Down Hour when you wake. Keep your phone on airplane mode in the morning, and don't take it off until after you have stretched, perhaps meditated and then had a moment to quietly eat breakfast.

61

MAKE SOME EMPTY SPACE

'Fill your bowl to the brim
and it will spill.
Keep sharpening your knife
and it will blunt.
Chase after money and security
and your heart will never unclench.
Care about people's approval
and you will be their prisoner.'

→ LAO TZU, PHILOSOPHER

In the ancient philosophy of Taoism, living your life in alignment is called The Great Way, or The Path. Our current cultural conditioning tells us that we must always fill our bowls to the brim, accumulating far more than we need. Even after we have all we need, we continue to acquire more and more. We reach for more approval and accolades and acknowledgement. There's no other species on earth that does this like humans do.

Today, I want you to notice where you're overfilling your metaphorical bowl, or blunting your symbolic knife. For example, are you pushing yourself too hard with exercise?

Are you working too many hours? Are you obsessed with productivity, but not actually producing anything? Are you meditating aggressively — just doing it to tick a box — or are you softening into your meditation practice, sitting and being present? Where are you overwhelming yourself with too many demands and too much expectation, and not being kind to yourself?

Let today be a day of softness and respect for yourself and others.

I'm not talking about getting rid of everything, but just gently paring things back. Have a look at the various parts of your day. Are you eating enough? Are you oversleeping? When your alarm goes off, do you just keep hitting snooze over and over again? Are you drinking too much caffeine? Are you overstimulating yourself? Today, be aware of what you're feeling, and just take it back a notch.

Have a beautiful day.

DAY 3

reduce
mashing

*stop multi-tasking
and be more
mindful*

'When you multi-task, you believe you're being exceptionally productive, but really, you're fooling yourself.'

→ KAREN FINERMAN, BUSINESSWOMAN

___

mind cleanse meditation
power down hour
$\rightarrow$ *reduce mashing*
morning ritual
banish busy
mind nutrition
joy ride

We don't need more time management; we need energy management. And the things that deplete our energy, such as being distracted and multi-tasking, must be eliminated. Mashing (aka multi-tasking) is when we do more than one thing at a time. It is now our way of life, mainly because we're so damn busy and our attention spans have become unbearably short.

> driving the car + speaking on the phone
  (hands-free, of course!) = mashing

> lying in bed + chatting to your partner
  + checking Pinterest = mashing

> talking to your kids + checking Instagram
  + paying for the groceries = mashing

> relaxing in the sun + reading a magazine
  + flicking through Facebook = mashing

> cooking dinner + listening to music
  + checking emails + shoving a load of
  washing into the machine = mashing

> going for a walk + taking a work phone call
  + sending yourself a 'reminder' email to
  take care of something later = mashing

67

The act of mashing robs us of actually experiencing what is happening. It means that we are never fully present and that we cannot pick up on the subtleties of each moment. Our instincts don't kick in, because we're never quite listening and we move from task to task in a blur.

We all have 24 hours in a day. It's what we eliminate and what we focus on that counts.

How do you manage this? Notice when you're mashing, and cut it out. Come to terms with the fact that you will never really do anything properly if you do everything all at once. Live in the moment, doing one thing at a time, and give each task all your attention. Remember: you're zapping yourself during peak times when you mash.

REDUCE MASHING

Sit down with a piece of paper and a pen, and quiet your mind and body. Slow your breathing. Rest a minute. Bring your awareness to how calm you feel when you are present.

Now scan the past week or two, and think of anything you mashed together. When did you attempt to increase your productivity in a way that likely just slowed you down? Acknowledge that you know you're not at your best when you do X and Y together. Notice the feeling in your body and mind as you are thinking about this chaotic approach, of mashing different tasks.

Write a list of things you know that you are mashing. I want you to be really honest with yourself. For whatever reason, you may have automatically wired together certain tasks. The intention usually seems logical, but the action of mashing is nonetheless wearing us down, fraying us, and making us distracted and fatigued.

When you finish your list, pin it up somewhere visible. For the rest of your 14 Day Mind Cleanse, keep it top of mind. Catch yourself mid-mash and stop immediately. Pause, smile and then just attend to one task at a time. A single action done well with your full attention is so much more fulfilling.

69

ACHIEVE TOTAL PRESENCE

There's an ancient Zen story about a monk who wanted to study with an older, very esteemed monk. The older monk refused to mentor him until he did a certain amount of training first. This training ended up taking many decades. Finally, the now not-so-young monk completed his studies and travelled three days to see the older monk at his small monastery up in the hills. When he arrived, it was pouring with rain. He shook himself off, folded his umbrella, removed his clogs and entered the small hall where the head monk was waiting. He sat in front of him and began to explain all the training he had done: six years in southern Japan, a decade with an esteemed monk in northern Japan, a few years here, a few more years there.

The older monk waited patiently until he had finished talking and then asked, 'On the way in, it was raining, yes?' The younger monk nodded. The older monk then asked, 'On which side of your clogs did you place your umbrella, left or right?' The younger monk looked baffled and conceded that he couldn't quite remember. The older monk calmly and gently replied, 'Still much Zen training to be done.'

Time and again, we get caught in the intellectual pursuits of self-development or spirituality and miss the foundations. The whole point is to be present in our lives, to live every moment of them clearly and in alignment with our higher selves. Too often this is missed when we delve into tricky philosophies or practices, when the fact is that every moment of our lives is part of our training! It doesn't just happen in the yoga studio, or on retreat, or listening to Tony Robbins or Tim Ferriss hype us up about life hacks.

Today, I want you to try paying attention to the here and now. Rather than fretting about the thing that you did an hour ago, or the thing that you must do later, really focus your attention on the present moment. How does your coffee taste, and what does it feel like as it swishes around your mouth? Can you feel the temperature of your tea through the cup you are holding? What does the water in your shower smell like as it trickles down over your body? How does every muscle, every limb, of your body feel as you dry yourself with the towel? Is the towel a little bit crispy because it's just come off the washing line, or is it soft because it's been used for a couple of days? What does your pillow feel like? What does the outside breeze on your skin feel like? How does the texture of paper feel when you pick it up? What is the sound of your knife and fork hitting the ceramic plate? Really dive into each experience today, and relish it. Imagine that today is your last day to enjoy what it means to be a human on earth, before you leave the planet forever. So, you want to suck as much out of each moment as possible.

Throughout the rest of the 14 Day Mind Cleanse, carry your attention – beautiful, pure and clean – with you into every moment of each day. On which side of the clogs did you place your umbrella? Can you recall it minutes or even hours later?

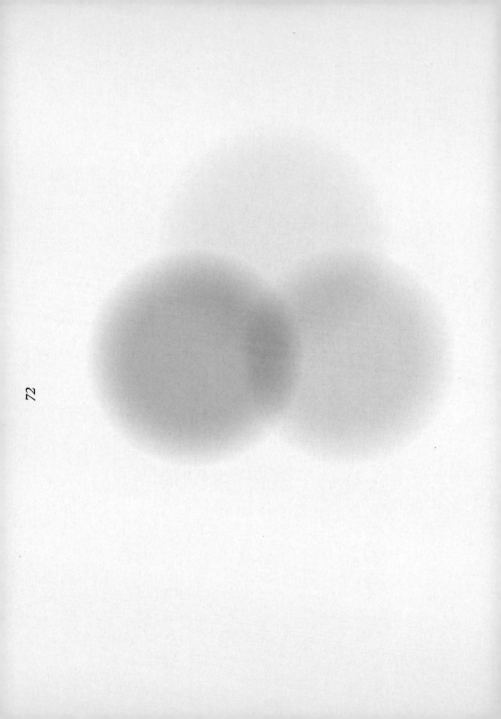

QUICK CHECK-IN

So you're on Day 3 now, and likely feeling the momentum of having committed to this program and putting yourself and your clarity first. Take it slowly, and give yourself a lot of space in which to process all that you're learning.

DAY 4

morning
ritual

*create a sequence
that upgrades
your whole day*

'When you arise in the morning, think of what a precious privilege it is to be alive – to breathe, to think, to enjoy, to love.'

→ MARCUS AURELIUS, EMPEROR OF ROME

mind cleanse meditation
power down hour
reduce mashing
→ morning ritual
banish busy
mind nutrition
joy ride

Sadhana is the Sanskrit term for daily practice or ritual. It is a spiritual practice where we bring our more present selves to the activity. There is a Zen saying that goes: 'When chopping wood, chop wood. When boiling water, boil water.' It means be reverent to every task; don't reserve being your best and most present self just for the 'special things', but for every moment in life.

The goal of *Sadhana* is to enable you to recover your natural rhythms and realign your inner life and daily habits with the cycles of the universe. When you begin to live and move with the rhythms of nature, your mind becomes more lucid and peaceful, and your health improves. Your entire life becomes easier.

Life is actually a series of micro choices. In this continuum of little moments, we make small decisions that either move us in the direction we wish to go, or pull us further into chaos and overwhelm. It's architecture with a schedule. This gentle daily discipline of adhering to a routine means that our creative minds can be freed up to focus on the important things. Often we mistakenly think that creativity is about chaos and spontaneity.

However, in order for us to be clear, creative and conscious, we need to create a platform of organization from which our days function.

Much attention has been given to the concepts of daily routine and practice. Celebrities and entrepreneurs are often quizzed about their habits as we attempt to unlock the ideal daily practice that will set us up for success. Steve Jobs reportedly employed an almost religious approach to routine and productivity. In a biography of the late Apple CEO, Walter Isaacson states that Jobs 'would pick four or five things that were really important for him to focus on and then just filter out – almost brutally – filter out the rest'. Author Haruki Murakami wakes at 4 am each day to work for a solid six hours, then exercises strenuously, and is in bed by 9 pm every night. Such diligence, he says, is the only way he can maintain physical strength and artistic sensitivity. I love this idea deeply. It doesn't work for me as I have a young family, but it is inspiration for the future.

MORNING RITUAL

Which activity nourishes you each day? What brings out the best in you? Is there something you wish you did every day but somehow don't find the time to do? Now is the time to introduce a ritual to your morning.

A structured and consistent morning ritual will provide you with a solid grounding for the day ahead. Maybe it's waking up 30 minutes earlier in the morning, so you don't rush around and take a pushed and panicky feeling into the rest of the day. Other activities you could choose include:

> take a brisk walk

> cuddle your cat

> drink a cup of tea or coffee quietly

> read a book

> have a bath

> eat a healthy breakfast

> stretch your muscles

> perform tai chi or yoga movements.

Grab a piece of paper or a notebook. Map out a potential morning ritual and the time you can dedicate to it. Ensure that it's just one thing and that it's doable every day. Then implement your ritual with flexibility and curiosity over the rest of your 14 Day Mind Cleanse.

This one commitment can make a huge difference when it is followed through with presence and detail. However, remember that in order to bring about a new routine, compassion must be employed or we set ourselves up for failure.

SET INTENTIONS

Mornings are also a powerful time to set intentions. These are signals to the brain and higher self about what the focus is for the day. Intention is the answer to gaining clarity and following through with action.

The important thing about intentions is that they are fluid and dynamic in nature. Don't become rigidly attached to them; accept that if they don't serve the need of the time, you can alter and change them. They can be upgraded if necessary.

Intentions benefit not only us, but also the greater good.
I read a beautiful little tale about a man who was standing on the seashore in the early morning, throwing starfish that had washed ashore back into the sea. Another man walked up to him and questioned his reason for doing this. The first man replied that if they stayed on the sand, they would dry up and die when the sun rose high in the sky. With a dismissive tone, the second man said he was being ridiculous and exclaimed, 'With the millions of starfish and the huge expanse of the ocean, how do you think you're ever going to make a difference?' The first man picked up another starfish, paused and replied, 'Well, I'm making a difference to this one,' as he threw it far into the water. This shows that our actions don't always need to be grandiose — but our intentions can be. When we serve others and not just ourselves, the reward is great.

While you are practicing your morning ritual, try setting an intention, or theme, for the day. It might be something like:

> Today I will be graceful.
> Today I will eat slowly and mindfully.
> Today I will focus on one task at a time.

Define your intention, and let everything stem from that.

DAY 5

**banish
busy**

*prioritize attention,
not activity*

'If you don't like something, change it. If you can't change it, change your attitude.'

→ MAYA ANGELOU, POET

mind cleanse meditation
power down hour
reduce mashing
morning ritual
→ *banish busy*
mind nutrition
joy ride

Every day is brimming with moments. And each moment is filled with feelings. These moments make up our hours, which make up our days, which fill our weeks and become months and, in turn, years. And we get to decide what we feel in each moment. Have you ever looked at your calendar and said, 'I cannot believe it's JUNE! Where is the year going?' Do you feel like life is going too fast, that you can't keep up? There is a solution. SLOW. IT. DOWN. You're the only one who can do this. Appreciate every moment – even the tough, tricky or uncomfortable ones – as they each hold learning. Cherish the charming, the joyous, the engaging and the funny. Relish them all.

You can't change time passing, but you can change your perspective on it.

We're going to shift our perspective on time, and what we do with it, to create more happiness and relaxation in each moment and in each day. Would you rather be stressed or relaxed? If you would love to live your days relaxed AND incredibly productive, then read on.

Let's take a look at a chunk of time. I want you to compare how it feels to spend 20 minutes doing each of the following:

> scrolling social media on a Sunday afternoon
> sitting in traffic, running late for a meeting
> meditating
> waiting at the hospital on test results
> dozing in the sun at the beach on a holiday
> writing emails in between meetings in a taxi
> lying in your lover's arms in bed before
  you have to get up and go to work.

I think you'll agree that they are all different kinds of time, and they can pass either very quickly or agonizingly slowly.

When we look at a week, with 24 hours in each day, we have 168 glorious hours at our disposal. The working week is usually 38 hours, but with overtime many people work for 50 hours a week. With eight hours of sleep a night, we are left with 62 hours a week where we are not sleeping or working. Let's take out another hour each day for eating and bathroom breaks. Now we have 55 free hours a week. What are we doing with that time?

Many of us have become modern masters of unproductivity.

Why are some people frantically busy, and others are chilled out and relaxed? How are some people accomplishing more and more, while others seem to get less and less done? And does our state of mind reflect our productivity and happiness?

BANISH BUSY

How many tasks and activities do you do every day? Ten? Forty? More? Does each day feel like a constantly evolving and growing list that spills into the next day?

Most days, we feel challenged by what we have to fit in, by work and by personal responsibilities. Part of trying to overcome this overwhelm is creating 'busyness' to ensure that we feel like we're achieving things. So we start by tackling the smaller and more manageable tasks first. We work on the insignificant things so that we can start ticking some boxes on our ever-growing list of tasks. And then we take a little break from the overwhelm by checking social media and our phones. After this mini break – otherwise known as a distraction – we get straight back to being busy again. Does your work pattern reflect this to a certain degree?

Having more time on your hands to savour life sounds wonderful, doesn't it? But we usually live in a way that's more 'daily grind' than 'making us happy'. The only person responsible for your own happiness and version of success is you. So what are you going to do about it? Buck the busy trend and do less – much less – each and every day.

For today and every remaining day of the 14 Day Mind Cleanse, I want you to choose the top three things you need to do. Focus on essential tasks, rather than the smaller and more menial ones. Then, after those top three vital things are achieved, assess whether you need to continue. Imagine if at midday, before lunch, you had all your important work out of the way. During the rest of the day — especially the afternoon crash period — you could relax because the day's difficult tasks had been done.

Think of yourself as a gallery owner, curating a show. What you choose to keep and what gets culled can result in a meaningful show or an unbalanced show that no one really enjoys. Treat every day like this. Quietly curate which tasks stay, and which don't. Think of each day as a meaningful experience, and not something that just has to be survived.

By doing less, you will be less stressed. It's madness to think that we can successfully tackle the many tasks we pop down on our to-do lists, and that the lists will ever be static — that no one will add responsibilities and tasks to our lists.

The only way to decrease your stress around your list is to ask yourself the hard questions and to prioritize the work. Does something actually need to be done, by you, today? By doing less, you can achieve more, as you focus on the important, meaningful work and not on the smaller, inconsequential tasks. By doing less, you can feel calmer, grounded and more in control. You're taking command of what's important to you in your day, and the rest can either wait or be left alone.

People focus on cramming in as much as they can, without being concerned with the quality. Doing one thing well means that you are present for that task, and you don't have to redo it. Less is more when it comes to quality productivity.

REFRAME 'BUSY'

'Busy' is a toxic word. It is everyone's standard go-to response for everything. We're all *sooooo* busy, all the time. However, what does busy really mean? I think it is code for: 'I am not prioritizing things in the right order. I am feeling overwhelmed and not being honest with you or myself about it.' But here's the thing: your brain registers whatever you say, whether it is fact or fiction, as your REALITY.

You will believe whatever you say in your mind. So when you say you're 'busy' all the time, your brain feels overwhelmed and exhausted. And when our brains are overwhelmed and exhausted, so are our bodies. Let's face it: we live in a modern world. We all have lots going on!

Try banning the phrase 'I am busy'. Reframing is where we consciously opt to think or say something else instead, to rewire our responses to situations and to employ a new attitude. It doesn't mean the first statement isn't true; it's just that we choose to highlight something else in its place. So rather than saying 'I am busy' all the time, experiment with phrases such as:

> 'I am engaged in some exciting projects.'
> 'I am challenged and inspired.'
> 'I have a lot on my plate at the moment.'
> 'I am certainly achieving a lot.'
> 'I am feeling full of purpose.'
> 'I am grateful for all of the good things I have going on in my life.'

Simplicity and focus are the keys to overcoming busy. The 14 Day Mind Cleanse is the process of cleaning out and cleaning up your thinking. Rewiring our brains can be challenging work, but it's worth it for the incredible results of ultra-focused, present, clear and decisive days.

QUICK CHECK-IN

Day 5! How are you feeling? What do you think is working the best for you so far? What is the most challenging? It's okay to find one technique more difficult than the others. Just keep going with the 14 Day Mind Cleanse; place one foot in front of the other.

DAY 6

mind
nutrition

*feed your mindset
and create better
emotional health*

'When intelligent people read, they ask themselves a simple question: What do I plan to do with this information?'

→ RYAN HOLIDAY, AUTHOR

mind cleanse meditation
power down hour
reduce mashing
morning ritual
banish busy
$\rightarrow$ *mind nutrition*
joy ride

We spend an unprecedented amount of time on technology. This evolution has happened at warp speed. Humans have been around for an incredibly long time, yet within a few short decades technology has become our major source of communication and our means of doing work, organizing our lives, buying groceries and banking.

I don't need to expound the effects of technology on all of us. There are some perks, of course. But is anyone actually stopping there? Are we only engaging with it for the sheer essentials? Of course not. Even grandmas and grandpas aren't just chatting to their grandkids on the iPad; they're also scrolling away, liking, adding friends, keeping in touch with siblings, playing games and reading the news. Technology has become all-consuming. Therefore, in the current age, retraining our brains on how they interact with technology is not just necessary – it's vital.

So today's focus is about proactively reducing mind waste and nourishing your mind every day for better mental health. Let's start by considering your Mind Nutrition. How healthy is the information you consume daily?

95

This includes conversations, news, social media, movies, TV series, books, magazines and blogs. Is it nourishing you and helping you grow? Or is it the information equivalent of a fizzy drink: sugary, caffeinated and with no nutritional value?

We need to consider our minds as we do our bodies, and fill them with healthy, inspiring and creative content.

Your happiness, clarity and creativity will all increase in proportion to your Mind Nutrition. So pay attention to where you can increase your consumption of healthy content, and what you might 'diet' or 'detox' out.

Now let's up the ante by addressing social media. Do you know what's social? Chatting to a friend over a coffee, or saying 'hi' to people at a party. Social media is awesome, and I love it – but social media is not social. Rather, it is a means by which we can carefully curate the perception other people have of our lives.

Are you someone who wakes up, turns off your alarm and instantly checks your Instagram? Then flicks over to email to see what came through overnight? Before hopping over to Facebook for five minutes, then relaxing back with your Instagram feed? All before you have even put your feet on your bedroom floor? I know this routine, as this was me.

My husband and I used to spend 'quality' time lying in bed together in the mornings, scrolling through social media. I knew this wasn't healthy behavior. But I was so addicted that I just couldn't stop. Something had to be done, so I came up with a set of rules. I turned off all of the notifications within each app, so my phone wasn't constantly harassing me, and I limited myself to checking social media only once a day. Like any detox program, I thought the withdrawal process would be painful. But instead it was INCREDIBLY LIBERATING.

MIND NUTRITION

Starting today and for the rest of your 14 Day Mind Cleanse, follow these three social-media rules:

1 Turn off all notifications.
2 Only check social media once or twice a day. Sit down to do this. Don't scroll in line at the grocery store, while waiting for a friend or when you are bored.
3 Set aside some time to stop following anyone who doesn't:
   – inspire you
   – enhance you
   – enliven you.

No more jealousy, not-good-enough feelings or excuses that 'they'll be upset if I don't follow them'.

You can go back to your normal ways after the 14 Day Mind Cleanse ends, although I doubt you will if you realize that you were addicted to social media.

97

ADD MORE POSITIVITY

Mind Nutrition isn't only about curating the information you consume, it's also about how you communicate to yourself. We don't want to fake being positive, but we also need to recognise that continual negativity serves absolutely no one. You're in charge of how you think, how you show up and how you communicate. There is so much talk about the power of positive thinking, so much science to back it up, yet I feel that most of us skim through and never really engage with it. Sometimes it feels too forced, or phoney, or as if we are kidding ourselves.

If you keep floundering around, saying 'I can't' through clenched teeth (and mind), then you will reinforce that exact thinking to your brain. If one human can do something, then so can another. And in reality, we have no idea what the billions of people in the world are up to. So there's really no excuse to think we can't do anything.

Take a little of this positivity into each day and see how things shift. You may have heard of the universal law of attraction. 'Like attracts like' and all that? The basic premise is that the more you have of one thing, the more you increase it. In other words, if you're being positive, even in the face of things going wrong, you will attract more positivity.

Think back to a day when it seemed like one thing after another went wrong. First, a flat tyre perhaps. Then you ran late for a major meeting, which made your boss angry, and the day just got progressively worse and worse. Now, think of another day, when everything seemed to go perfectly. No traffic, you nailed each meeting, you got along with everyone, and you were in an incredible mood.

While external events are out of your control, the world will also keep reflecting back to you the way you perceive things to be. Joy means more joy. Frustration equates to more frustration.

The good news is that you can master these outcomes. Being positive is important in order to attract more positivity. Today and for the rest of your 14 Day Mind Cleanse, if you catch yourself in the middle of negative thinking, put a handbrake on that thought. Replace it by silently saying something positive to yourself. For example:

> Replace focusing on your weaknesses with thinking about your many strengths.
> Replace focusing on how others view you with how you view yourself.
> Replace focusing on what you don't have with what you currently do have.

Be aware of your self-talk. Don't say things to yourself that you wouldn't say to a child or a close friend. **Reinforce your positive thinking with positive language.**

LEAVE THE WEEDS

There's an old Sufi story about a man who decided to start a flower garden. He prepared the soil and planted the seeds of many beautiful flowers, but when the plants grew, his garden was filled with not just his chosen flowers but also dandelion weeds. He sought out advice from experts and tried every known method to get rid of the weeds, but to no avail. Finally, he walked all the way to the capital city to converse with the head gardener, who suggested a variety of remedies to expel the dandelions. But the man had already tried them all. They sat together in silence for some time. Finally, the head gardener looked at him and said, 'Well, then I suggest you learn to love them.'

100

What are the 'dandelions' in your life at the moment? What are the things you've been trying to reduce or get rid of, and how might you learn to love them? Maybe it's part of your job, or a person in your life, or an annoying situation. How might you soften into and learn to love that thing, that person, that behavior, that action, so you can start to move forward with more grace?

This definitely doesn't mean that you should no longer set boundaries, but that there are some situations in which — as with the gardener — we've tried everything to no avail. It's very important for our Mind Nutrition that we learn how to love in these situations.

As you contemplate the weeds in your life, I recommend journalling about them. Where are the weeds in your work life, in your relationships and within yourself? What are the things that you can't reconcile about yourself? What are the stories you keep telling yourself, the personal weeds you keep trying to rip out? Can you learn to love them as well? It's important to remember that some things in life cannot be worked through without professional help, such as the care of a psychologist. So go gently, and if you feel like you need additional help, seek a professional to guide you through this process.

Sometimes we can spend too much time trying to pull out the weeds — if we just let them be or even gave them a little love, they might sort themselves out on their own. You can pay attention to all of the beautiful flowers — enriching your mind — or you can continue to put all your energy into dealing with the weeds. Which will you choose?

DAY 7

joy ride

*increase
your happiness
and positivity*

'We cannot cure the world of sorrows, but we can choose to live in joy.'

→ JOSEPH CAMPBELL, AUTHOR

mind cleanse meditation
power down hour
reduce mashing
morning ritual
banish busy
mind nutrition
$\rightarrow$ *joy ride*

Remember that episode of *The Simpsons* where Marge blew a mind gasket and froze up on the bridge, windows up, refusing to come out of the car? She was so overwhelmed by responsibility and the lack of time to herself that she just lost it. It's scary to stand on the edge of such an emotional cliff.

Carving out some aloneness – the space to breathe and meditate – is imperative.

We need time to cultivate ideas, feel through concepts and simply be as a human being instead of constantly engaging with the world.

In today's frantic age, I think it should be one of our greatest commitments. Because peaceful people who know themselves and don't feel besieged usually act kindly and with compassion, and don't do a lot of the awful things that we are capable of as humans. So let's stop feeling guilty for taking some moments for ourselves.

Everything we experience, emotionally or physically, is the result of chemical reactions in our bodies. These reactions are responsible for negative feelings and experiences, but they are also the reason for our joy and positivity. Love, happiness, compassion: these are all the result of a bunch of hormones that, when in balance, come to the rescue in times of need.

Endorphins, serotonin, dopamine and oxytocin are what we call the 'happy hormones'. They help us have a higher tolerance to pain and physical stress, they regulate mood, and they prevent depression, making us happy and sociable. They guide us in the direction of love and are the reason we strive towards our goals and feel satisfied and accomplished when we reach them.

Of course, all of our hormones are designed to work in harmony, so we don't necessarily want an overabundance of these happy hormones, as that can lead to hard crashes, moments of feeling abandoned and loss of trust. This is what tends to happen when we lean on substances such as alcohol or drugs to provide these feelings. What we want is balance and to let our bodies move with their natural rhythms. When we are in this state of balance, we are able to sit in the discomfort of a rough time, and grow and be present in positive moments.

JOY RIDE

While things such as promotions, marriage, buying a house and the birth of your children are incredible, they are also rare events that we can't experience all the time. If we postpone our happiness and joy to the weekend, or a holiday, or that promotion, we are literally robbing ourselves of an enormous amount of happiness and joy that's there waiting for us, every single day.

Happiness shouldn't be some far-off goal. It should be a daily reality. And it can be, when we remember that it's the little things in life that bring us the most joy. This exercise is going to ensure that you feel happiness and joy every day.

Grab a pen and paper, sit down and get ready to get stuck in. Write down ten small things that make you happy. Focus on little events or activities that are UNIQUE to you. Holidays and birthdays are common to everyone, so they don't make the list.

This should be a list of happiness-inducing activities that occupy a special little place in your soul, and that are part of what makes you who you are. My list includes:

> drinking a hot cup of tea in the morning, and eating toast with an obscene amount of salted butter
> sleeping in when it rains

> reading cookbooks, and cooking with beautiful produce
> fumbling about in our ramshackle garden at home
> watching the sunrise
> taking long walks with my husband on a quiet weekend, when we talk about our lives
> devouring non-fiction books.

What's on your list?

Now look closely at your list and think about how many of the activities you ACTUALLY do on a regular basis. Each day? Each week? Each month? You might be surprised to discover that although these simple-yet-awesome things bring you so much happiness, you're hardly doing them at all.

These items are your 'joy rides'. Today and every day during the rest of the 14 Day Mind Cleanse, you are going to do at least one of them. These are simple keys to unlocking more joy and happiness in your life. It sounds easy, right? But it can be a challenge.

Put the list up on your fridge, beside your bed or above your desk at work as a reminder to keep your joy rides up after the end of the 14 Day Mind Cleanse.

If you are looking at your list and realising that you're already engaging with some of these joy rides, then this is fabulous. Be even more ambitious with prioritizing your joy.

You are responsible for your own happiness and joy. Yes, you. No one else.

GIVE UP COMPLAINING

In his book *Awareness*, Anthony de Mello — one of my favorite spiritual teachers — wrote about happiness. (I highly recommend you listen to this as an audio book, because Anthony's voice is just so beautiful and charismatic.) He noted that **we all have happiness within us; the only thing in the way of us experiencing happiness is the fact that we have negative conditioning, ideas and illusions.** And if we just let those go, then we would experience an abundance of happiness, joy and high vibes. So why is letting them go so insanely challenging?

I want to run a little experiment with you today. Try to pause your complaining throughout the day. Complaining is so easy and enticing to do. We whip out our little imaginary violins and play a sad song called 'Woe Is Me', which completely undermines our happiness, our clarity and our creativity. As Anthony notes, we have to DROP SOMETHING to feel happiness. So for today (and hopefully in the future), that something will be complaining.

Become aware of how attached you are to complaining. It's a worshipping of our problems. In the philosophy of Vedanta, the practice of Tapasya is giving up something in order to gain something else for a period of time. The first time I did Tapasya, I let go of coffee, which for me was a really big deal. But rather than not drinking coffee for three months and then using my tension around this as a way to soften what I did, I became very melodramatic about it all. I would refer to it at every opportunity. If I was fatigued, I would say to someone, 'Oh, I'm so tired, but it's because I'm not drinking coffee.' I would go to a coffee shop and order a tea, but have to tell the barista that I would love a latte but wasn't drinking coffee, and go on and on about it. This wasn't the path to happiness or to gaining awareness about my attachments. And somewhat ironically, I was complaining about my Tapasya. It was actually the path to being really melodramatic and engaged in my own drama.

I want you to be really aware today (and over the rest of the 14 Day Mind Cleanse, but particularly today) of where you are getting stuck on your complaining. How can you bring joy and lightness to the situations you view as challenging? Eventually, you will start to ask yourself some deep questions:

> What am I really attached to here?
> Why am I so stuck on complaining about my life?
> What are the real mechanics behind the complaining?
> What is my conditioning?
> What is my illusion around why I think I need to whine about this thing so desperately?

Complaining is a bit of a blind spot for most of us. By consciously pausing our complaining, there is more space to experience happiness and joy about the good things in our lives. Where attention goes, energy flows!

QUICK CHECK-IN

You've completed your first week! How are you feeling at this point? How are you doing emotionally? As with any detox, there can be some dramatic feelings and sometimes you can be a bit unsettled. All is well, though, as this is a natural part of the process. You're quite literally rewiring your brain and mind! Be patient with yourself. This is why we have another week to stabilize your learning and dive deeper into the benefits.

WEEK 2

deep cleanse

'Put your heart, mind, and soul into even your smallest acts. This is the secret of success.'

→ SWAMI SIVANANDA, HINDU SPIRITUAL TEACHER

mind cleanse meditation
power down hour
reduce mashing
morning ritual
banish busy
mind nutrition
joy ride
$\rightarrow$ *journalling*

Congratulations on completing your first week of the 14 Day Mind Cleanse. We'll now take a second week to put all of the techniques into practice for a deep cleanse. Your brain has done a lot of learning this past week, and now it is time to settle in and see the benefits.

As a reminder, listed above is your full 'menu' of Mind Cleanse building-block techniques to be repeated each day for days 8 to 14. For this second week, we'll also add a journalling activity, with a set of prompts for you to reflect upon each evening.

The journalling might take you just a few minutes, or you might spend more time digesting your experience of the day and really diving in. You're welcome to write in the spaces provided in this book or to use a separate notebook. I always love to have special notebooks and journals for my recollections, thoughts and ideas. So if you feel like splurging, get something lovely to write in.

Documenting your processes and feelings is a way to remind your brain of what has happened, and to wire in your learning and experiences.

It helps with cognitive change and can be a really creative process. Remember, no one is going to read this! It's just for you. If you're not familiar with journalling, the first day or so can feel a little strange – but it will gain more flow as you go.

Ideally, do the journalling in your evening Power Down Hour, so you have no digital distractions and can really settle into writing about the day. It will soon become a much-loved ritual that you are likely to continue for years to come.

Week 2 overview

Each day you will complete all seven techniques from Week 1, as well as a journalling exercise. This is what you will do every day during Week 2:

mind cleanse meditation

power down hour

reduce mashing

morning ritual

banish busy

mind nutrition

joy ride

journalling

DAY 8

FOLLOW THE FULL MIND CLEANSE MENU (SEE PAGE 117). AT THE END OF THE DAY, REFLECT ON YOUR EXPERIENCE AND WRITE YOUR ANSWERS TO THE FOLLOWING:

Which technique did you find the most helpful for you today?

What is one thing that you learned about yourself today? *Explore an extension from this, such as what you will do about this moving forward. For example, if you learned that the Power Down Hour is challenging with your phone nearby, your learning is to keep it out of the room.*

Did you feel present or distracted today? When, and why?

How did you find your meditation practice? *Avoid saying 'good' or 'bad' and instead use adjectives such as calm, choppy, long and dreamy.*

Write about three things that you're grateful to have experienced today. *These can be large things or something as simple as the sun on your face or a phone call with a friend.*

DAY 9

FOLLOW THE FULL MIND CLEANSE MENU (SEE PAGE 117).
AT THE END OF THE DAY, REFLECT ON YOUR EXPERIENCE
AND WRITE YOUR ANSWERS TO THE FOLLOWING:

Which technique did you find the most helpful for you today?

What is one thing that you learned about yourself today? *Explore an
extension from this, such as what you will do about this moving forward.
For example, did you have a day that you spent being very 'busy'? How
might tomorrow look if you reframed that?*

Did you feel present or distracted today? When, and why?

How did you find your meditation practice?

Write about three things that you're grateful to have experienced today.

DAY 10

*FOLLOW THE FULL MIND CLEANSE MENU (SEE PAGE 117).
AT THE END OF THE DAY, REFLECT ON YOUR EXPERIENCE
AND WRITE YOUR ANSWERS TO THE FOLLOWING:*

Which technique did you find the most helpful for you today?

What is one thing that you learned about yourself today? *Explore an extension from this, such as what you will do about this moving forward. For example, how did you go with your joy-riding? How do you feel when you engage with activities that bring you joy?*

Did you feel present or distracted today? When, and why?

How did you find your meditation practice?

Write about three things that you're grateful to have experienced today.

DAY 11

FOLLOW THE FULL MIND CLEANSE MENU (SEE PAGE 117).
AT THE END OF THE DAY, REFLECT ON YOUR EXPERIENCE
AND WRITE YOUR ANSWERS TO THE FOLLOWING:

Which technique did you find the most helpful for you today?

What is one thing that you learned about yourself today? Explore an
extension from this, such as what you will do about this moving forward.
For example, how is your morning ritual shaping up? What are you
enjoying about it, and are there any tweaks that you can make to it?

Did you feel present or distracted today? When, and why?

How did you find your meditation practice?

Write about three things that you're grateful to have experienced today.

DAY 12

FOLLOW THE FULL MIND CLEANSE MENU (SEE PAGE 117). AT THE END OF THE DAY, REFLECT ON YOUR EXPERIENCE AND WRITE YOUR ANSWERS TO THE FOLLOWING:

Which technique did you find the most helpful for you today?

What is one thing that you learned about yourself today? *Explore an extension from this, such as what you will do about this moving forward. For example, what are you learning about yourself by reducing mashing? How do you feel when you catch yourself mashing too many tasks?*

Did you feel present or distracted today? When, and why?

How did you find your meditation practice?

Write about three things that you're grateful to have experienced today.

DAY 13

FOLLOW THE FULL MIND CLEANSE MENU (SEE PAGE 117). AT THE END OF THE DAY, REFLECT ON YOUR EXPERIENCE AND WRITE YOUR ANSWERS TO THE FOLLOWING:

Which technique did you find the most helpful for you today?

What is one thing that you learned about yourself today? *Explore an extension from this, such as what you will do about this moving forward. For example, did you find it difficult to reduce the time you spent feeding your mind with social media? How will you change your habits?*

Did you feel present or distracted today? When, and why?

How did you find your meditation practice?

Write about three things that you're grateful to have experienced today.

DAY 14

FOLLOW THE FULL MIND CLEANSE MENU (SEE PAGE 117). AT THE END OF THE DAY, REFLECT ON YOUR EXPERIENCE AND WRITE YOUR ANSWERS TO THE FOLLOWING:

Which technique did you find the most helpful for you today?

What is one thing that you learned about yourself today? Explore an extension from this, such as what you will do about this moving forward. It's the final day of your 14 Day Mind Cleanse! Today's learning might be a piece of wisdom you can carry forward for a long time.

Did you feel present or distracted today? When, and why?

How did you find your meditation practice?

Write about three things that you're grateful to have experienced today.

CONCLUSION

what a huge
two weeks!

Congratulations!

You made it, and have completed your 14 Day Mind Cleanse. Rewiring our brains – as well as acknowledging and working with our beliefs, our ingrained patterns and our habits – can be challenging at times, can't it? Transformation isn't always easy. However, no matter how easy or challenging you found the past fortnight, I hope that on completion you feel a sense of calm, as well as curiosity about how you might continue with the elements that really worked for you.

You have worked through philosophies and techniques, and have brought new practices into your life. At the beginning of this book, I asked you to think about why you were undertaking this Mind Cleanse. Now I ask you this: do you still feel that the same reasons apply? Or did the process itself give you more clarity as to why you took it on?

I also asked you about your level of commitment to bringing more clarity into your life. Do you feel that you really gave yourself the best shot you could to actualize this? What can you learn from your approach? If you were to immediately do it again, how would you do it differently? Specifically, what would you NOT do, and what would you ensure that you did more of? For example, would you be more vigilant with each Power Down Hour and become more disciplined with putting down tech? Or could you have given something more time and energy, for example joy-riding?

And most importantly, how do you feel overall now?

Moving forward, I wanted to share some ideas and tips for continuing to engage with the 14 Day Mind Cleanse, by implementing the techniques that worked for you. Keep refining and customising the techniques over time as they become more and more familiar and part of your daily life. Additionally, come back and introduce – for a single week – a technique that you found really challenging. Often it's the techniques that we find the hardest that are the best for us, but we naturally shy away from the challenge and adopt the more easily integrated elements. Revisiting a single technique and working your way through it would be enormously helpful.

If you are ready to take your meditation practice up a level, I would love to see you learn Mindfit Meditation or Integrated Meditation. You can find out more at thebroadplace.com.

Lastly, you can revisit the 14 Day Mind Cleanse as a powerful reset tool for mind and brain whenever you feel foggy, overwhelmed or simply want more clarity and creativity in your life. You will learn something new every time you undertake the 14 Day Mind Cleanse, because you grow and evolve so much during the process and in the space between cleanses. Too often we are running on empty, experiencing burnout and exhaustion, and ignoring the simple, distilled things that work for us in our lives. So recognize when you're feeling mind fatigue or fog, and get on top of it early with these helpful techniques.

One more thing before we part: above all, I hope you learned that you are capable beyond what you might believe. I hope you learned that you are creative, clear and cognizant, but often stuck in habits that don't serve you, and that editing and pausing these – and introducing healthier ways of being – can be a much simpler process than you might have originally thought. I hope you feel empowered to continue. I hope you realize that by taking time for yourself – to meditate, journal, do the things that bring you joy, engage with present-moment awareness, pay attention and take care – you are ultimately more productive, and happier for it. And I hope you continue to learn, expand and grow.

With kindness,
Jac

HERE'S A JOURNALLING EXERCISE FOR YOU TO WRAP UP THE PROCESS.
WE WOULD ABSOLUTELY LOVE IT IF YOU WOULD SHARE YOUR ANSWERS
WITH US IN A SHORT SURVEY THAT WE HAVE CREATED FOR YOU AT
www.thebroadplace.com/14daymindcleanse.

Of all the techniques you learned, which one was the most valuable for you personally? Why? *(There's insight to be gained into which techniques will work for you in the future!)*

Which part did you find the most challenging, and why?

What was the most interesting learning or discovery that you made about yourself?

Which techniques will you continue now that you have completed the 14 Day Mind Cleanse?

How do you feel on conclusion, and what experiences do you want to continue to enhance?

RESOURCES

Here are a few of my other books, as well as a comprehensive list of the best titles in self-development and spirituality. I've also included some of the books that I have found personally life-changing, to help you align to your most clear, creative and confident self.

A Mind at Home with Itself: How asking four questions can free your mind, open your heart, and turn your world around by Byron Katie

The Art of Asking: Or how I learned to stop worrying and let people help by Amanda Palmer

Big Magic: Creative living beyond fear by Elizabeth Gilbert

Ego Is the Enemy: The fight to master our greatest opponent by Ryan Holiday

Falling into Grace: Insights on the end of suffering by Adyashanti

The Four Agreements: A practical guide to personal freedom by Don Miguel Ruiz

Four Thousand Weeks: Time and how to use it by Oliver Burkeman

Freedom from the Known by J. Krishnamurti

The Gifts of Imperfection: Let go of who you think you're supposed to be and embrace who you are by Brené Brown

Grist for the Mill: Awakening to oneness by Ram Dass

High Grade Living: A guide to creativity, clarity and mindfulness by Jacqui Lewis and Arran Russell

How to Cook Your Life: From the Zen kitchen to enlightenment by Dogen Zenji

Letters Edition One by Jacqui Lewis

Love for Imperfect Things: How to accept yourself in a world striving for perfection by Haemin Sunim

Make the Impossible Possible: One man's crusade to inspire others to dream bigger and achieve the extraordinary by Bill Strickland

Mothers Mind Cleanse: A handbook of philosophy and tools to be a calmer, happier mother in our modern world by Jacqui Lewis

My Stroke of Insight: A brain scientist's personal journey by Jill Bolte Taylor, PhD

No Bad Parts: Healing trauma & restoring wholeness with the Internal Family Systems model by Richard C. Schwartz, PhD

Power, Freedom and Grace: Living from the source of lasting happiness by Deepak Chopra

Real Estate by Deborah Levy

Rethink: The way you live by Amanda Talbot

She Wants It: Desire, power, and toppling the patriarchy by Jill Soloway

The Tao of Inner Peace by Diane Dreher

Tao Te Ching translated by Stephen Mitchell

The Untethered Soul: The journey beyond yourself by Michael A. Singer

The Way of Integrity: Finding the path to your true self by Martha Beck

The Wisdom of No Escape: How to love yourself and your world by Pema Chödrön

THANKS

I would like to thank the entire team at Murdoch Books for their truly inspiring efforts with this project, especially the originating publisher, Kelly Doust. As a team, they were creative, diligent and so supportive, and it has made the process of bringing this book to life one of my favorites to date.

Jane Novak, my literary agent, deserves huge thanks. I am so grateful for her unlimited belief in this book and in me.

I would like to thank my wonderful husband, Arran Russell. He is still my favorite human to date and an endlessly creative soundboard, collaborator and realist. There is no one who believes in my capacity to create and share more than him, and I will be forever in awe of his creativity and the way he shows up in the world, which inspires so much of who I am.

Thanks to my daughter, Marley, who patiently watches me undertake these enormous projects and sees the frustration, the joy, the discomfort and the pleasure they bring. I hope that continuing to see the creative process inspires her in her life.

I would also like to thank all of The Broad Place students. It's been an incredible, wild, bumpy, expansive and beautiful decade with all of our students from around the world, and without them, this book wouldn't even be possible. Thank you.

Quarto

This edition published in 2023 by Chartwell Books,
an imprint of The Quarto Group
142 West 36th Street, 4th Floor
New York, NY 10018 USA
T (212) 779-4972 F (212) 779-6058
www.Quarto.com

First published in 2018 by Murdoch Books, an imprint of Allen & Unwin

Murdoch Books Australia
83 Alexander Street,
Crows Nest NSW 2065
Phone: +61 (0)2 8425 0100
murdochbooks.com.au
info@murdochbooks.com.au

Murdoch Books UK
Ormond House, 26–27 Boswell Street,
London, WC1N 3JZ
Phone: +44 (0) 20 8785 5995
murdochbooks.co.uk
info@murdochbooks.co.uk

Publisher: Diana Hill
Editorial Manager: Jane Price
Design: Madeleine Kane
Editor: Kay Halsey
Photography: Phil Webb
Photographer's assistant: Simon Reed
Styling and food preparation: Jennifer Joyce assisted by Zoe Harrington
Illustrations: Riley Joyce
Production Director: Lou Playfair

ISBN 978-0-7858-4318-4

Colour reproduction by Splitting Image Colour Studio Pty Ltd, Clayton, Victoria

Printed in China.